Culinary Grief Therapy

Culinary Grief Therapy

COOKING-FOR-ONE SERIES

Heather Lynn Nickrand

Recipes Created By Laura Lerdal And David Kramer

AMITA Health Alexian Brothers Press

Published by AMITA Health Alexian Brothers Press
800 Biesterfield Rd
Elk Grove Village, IL 6007

ISBN-13: 9780692860694
ISBN-10: 069286069X

Dedication

This book is dedicated to all the people we had the true privilege of walking alongside with on this journey. Your compassion, dedication, and resilience put forth to rediscover a new sense of meaning, purpose, and happiness is truly remarkable. This book is dedicated to all of your hearts and connected with ours. We are here to walk this with you every step of the way–one step at a time.

Acknowledgments

The Cooking-for-One workshops could not have been possible without the compassionate participation of professional chefs Laura Lerdal and David Kramer. Their dedication and support is truly heartfelt and gratefully acknowledged. The recipes submitted are created with such care and professionalism for people who have lost a loved one. Our visions are shared and I am truly blessed with a wonderful partnership between AMITA Health Alexian Brothers Hospice and the College of Dupage Culinary and Hospitality Center.

To my family, friends, co-workers, clients, and others who in one way or another shared their support, thank you from the bottom of my heart. I am forever grateful.

Introduction

This complete skills workbook is directed at the general public, healthcare providers, and individuals and family members who have lost a loved one. The workbook contains grief exercises, healthy grieving techniques, recipes on cooking-for-one, and self-assessment strategies to be utilized at various stages for coping with daily life in adjusting to a new normal after loss.

This workbook provides help in weekly meal planning, preparing shopping lists, gauging portion size, and utilizing leftovers to create new meals with attention to personal milestones and holidays. Because leftovers can be painful reminders of missing loved ones, all recipes are designed to minimize food waste, with leftovers from previous meals being used in new recipes. *Culinary Grief Therapy* features grief exercises in guided recipe memoir writing, personal reflections, trigger identification, cognitive mapping, and guided meditation exercises. Drawn from cognitive behavioral therapy, objectives for the workbook are to correct negative thought patterns on meal planning to a relational journey of adaption to the loss in learning new strategies to meal plan, shop, and cook while enjoying meals at home without a loved one. This workbook can help you address irrational beliefs, feelings of depression or anger, and avoidance or numbing behaviors with a goal of leading to adapting to a life in cooking-for-one.

As part of the bereavement counseling program in AMITA Health Alexian Brothers Hospice, a need was identified by Heather Nickrand, MA, LPC, NCC in individuals who had lost loved ones and were having difficulty with adjusting to meal planning, shopping, and cooking-for-one. Individuals expressed feelings of loneliness and depression when grocery shopping and cooking for themselves alone, which led to many painful memories of the loss of their loved one. The feelings of grief lingered throughout the day and had a negative effect on subsequent meals leading to avoidance of activities, skipped meals, and unhealthy coping mechanisms. To address this need for grief counseling, *Culinary Grief Therapy: Cooking-for-One Series* was developed. The *Cooking-for-One Series* provides the components of a grief support group in a culinary setting.

Contents

CHAPTER 1

Coping Techniques for Grocery Shopping-for-One

Ten Steps for Healthy Coping Patterns after the Loss of a Loved One

- Have a Plan
- Measure Your Comfort Level
- Practice Relaxation, Deep Breathing, and Guided Mediation
- Make Lists
- Activate Your Task-Brain and Rest Your Grieving-Brain
- Select Colors First
- Ask for Help
- Use Grounding Exercises
- Learn Proportioning and Sizing
- Reward Yourself

Step One: Have a Plan

Going grocery shopping after the loss of a loved one requires a plan.

First and foremost, pick a grocery store that speaks to you. Though you may be tempted to go to an entirely new store, you should start your journey on terrain you feel comfortable with.

Selecting a familiar grocery store will allow you to normalize the setting and thus help reduce stress and anxiety. Once you have decided on your grocery store, you are halfway there—you've made the initial decision. Congratulate yourself! This process is all about baby steps.

Next take a moment to visualize the store you selected and all the elements in the store. It is best to complete this task somewhere peaceful and quiet. Begin by visualizing the outside of the store. Visualize the signs, the entrance, and the parking lot. Allow yourself to see everything.

Now visually step inside the store and take a look around. Be sure to use all your senses. Consider what you can see, what you can smell, what you can touch, what you can hear, and what you can taste. Next visualize the aisles. More importantly, take note of which aisles contain certain items and where those items are shelved. Then decide which path to start moving toward.

You should visually explore different aisles and paths depending on your mood and thoughts. There is no right or wrong way to do this. The best technique in selecting your path is to read your feelings and behaviors as they happen, without judgment.

Step Two: Measure Your Comfort Level

Take a moment to assess your basic comfort level. On a scale of 1–10 rate your level of comfort in shopping for one at the grocery store.

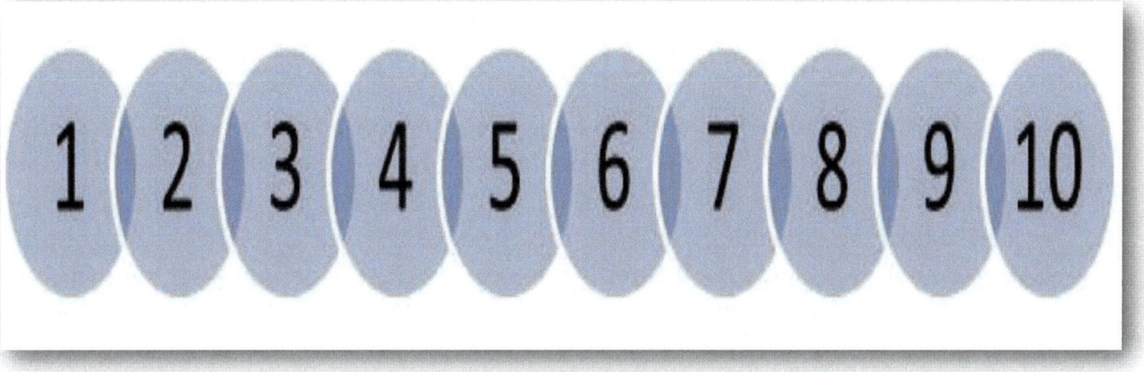

It is best to make this assessment in full honesty. This rating is a reading of your "grief temperature." There is no good or bad number. It is simply an indicator of how to approach this particular task of coping.

- **Rating of 1–3**
  If your score is in the 1–3 range, it is best to take a dry run of the grocery store initially. Simply take a drive to the grocery store. Do not go inside. You want to introduce the setting to your mind and body first in order to reduce the intensity of your response. Spend some time driving in the parking lot before you park, and then assess your comfort level. If you are feeling comfortable, continue to sit in the spot. If the weather is nice, roll down the windows and allow the fresh air to calm your nerves. Put on some pleasant music, or bring a book with you. The purpose of this exercise is to familiarize the person you are now with the grocery store and to understand what it means to be entering the grocery store as one. This part of the grieving process involves adjusting to a new normal and rediscovering a sense of meaning, purpose, and happiness. Give yourself the appropriate time to just sit and be present. Deep breathing is a very useful coping strategy in this stage.

- **Rating of 4–6**
  If your score is in the 4–6 range, it is best to practice mindful imagery. You can also pair mindful imagery with the dry run discussed in the previous section to effectively desensitize yourself and reduce the impact of the anxiety-inducing situation (going to the grocery store). Then, in order to reduce the fear of shopping-for-one, use relaxation techniques (such as deep breathing, meditation, listening to music, and reading) to obtain a calm and rational mind-set. Most important is to select a relaxation technique

that works for you, not for someone else. In addition, it is also very healthy to switch up relaxation techniques to avoid becoming stuck in the same cognitive processes.

- **Rating of 7–10**
  If your score is in the 7–10 range, such a score indicates that the individual already has found a way to effectively manage his or her grief and that those strategies and techniques should be continued. Journaling is a great tool to use at this level. In fact, journaling *throughout* the hierarchy allows you to reflect on your grief work and the strides you have taken. With grief, it is common to dismiss the steps already completed and focus solely on the steps still ahead. However, in order to get to where we are going, we need to take the time to reflect on where we have been and how we have progressed. Journaling is a wonderful tool for recording your progress. Rate your reactions in a journal each time you tackle the grocery store, taking note of similarities, patterns, triggers, and feelings.

It is important to note that these scores will change frequently, which means you should rate yourself more than once. How you feel will differ from day to day. Repeat this exercise to serve as checkpoints on your journey. Be kind to yourself, and meet yourself where you are today. Remember to journal often to keep track of your progress. It is also beneficial to share these exercises with loved ones and "safe people"—those you can trust with your grief and who understand what you are going through. Identifying your safe people is vital, but keep in mind that your safe people may not be the closest people in your inner circle. Although your safest person is no longer with you to hold your hand, sometimes you can find his or her hands through the hands of others. Give your reactions, responses, and experiences a place to be safely released instead of keeping them locked inside of you. Holding all of those emotions inside creates weight and resistance. It is the true release of our grieving experiences that allows us to take bigger steps and reach greater heights.

Step Three: Practice Relaxation, Deep Breathing, and Guided Meditation

Explanation of Deep Breathing

The purpose of meditation is to calm the mind, not to stop the mind entirely. Doing the latter creates difficulty in reaching a healthy meditated state. It is important to center your breathing patterns while you are grieving; otherwise your thoughts will control the rhythm of your breathing. More times than not, we follow our thoughts without paying any attention to our breath. Following your breath shifts the dynamic of control. You—not your thoughts—are in control of your breath. Additionally, engaging in calming breathing patterns throughout the day reduces intrusive thoughts and cycling questions and doubts.

This concept is similar to having a radio playing in the background while you engage in a task: your main focus is on the task at hand. Yes, you can hear the radio, but that does not stop you from, for example, doing the dishes. You are still able to pick up a plate, wash it, and dry it. The music is simply running in the background. In a deep-breathing exercise, the radio is your running thoughts while doing the dishes is the task. Make mindfulness (deep breathing) your task, and let the music from the radio (your thoughts) serve as distant background noise: take it in, but don't let it prevent you from completing your task. Let your running thoughts be present, but focus on your breath. Let your breath be in control.

As you practice deep breathing and controlling your breath, give your thoughts a source of direction. It is helpful to use a stress ball in practicing this skill. As you breathe, you squeeze. As you take a breath in, squeeze the stress ball, mirroring your breath. As you release the stress ball, release your breath. With faster breaths, make rapid squeezes. With deeper breaths, make calmer squeezes. If the breath is held, squeeze the ball and hold until *you* choose to release it. You are in full control of your decisions and the way you feel. Prevent your grief from controlling the ball by giving your thoughts a focus.

Guided Meditation Exercise

- Close your eyes and focus on your breath. Be aware of all body positions.
- Ask Yourself: Is the chair supporting you, or are you supporting the chair?
- Body Scan: Do you notice any pain or tension?
- Welcome any thoughts coming in, and then let them go, without judgment.
- What emotions are you feeling right now? Name those emotions.
- Welcome any emotions coming in, and then let them go, without judgment.
- Imagine a place you feel comfortable or safe, and picture that place. Use your senses to take you there.
- What do you see? What color is the sky or paint on the walls?
- What do you hear? Is there water rushing or laughter in the background?
- What do you taste? Is anything sweet or sour?
- What do you smell? Do you smell a favorite home-cooked meal or a specific scent?
- What do you feel? Do you feel anything cold, warm, or soft?
- Take a few more minutes and keep noticing all of your sesnes, focusing on where you are. When you are ready, slowly open your eyes and arrive back into the room.

Step Four: Make Lists

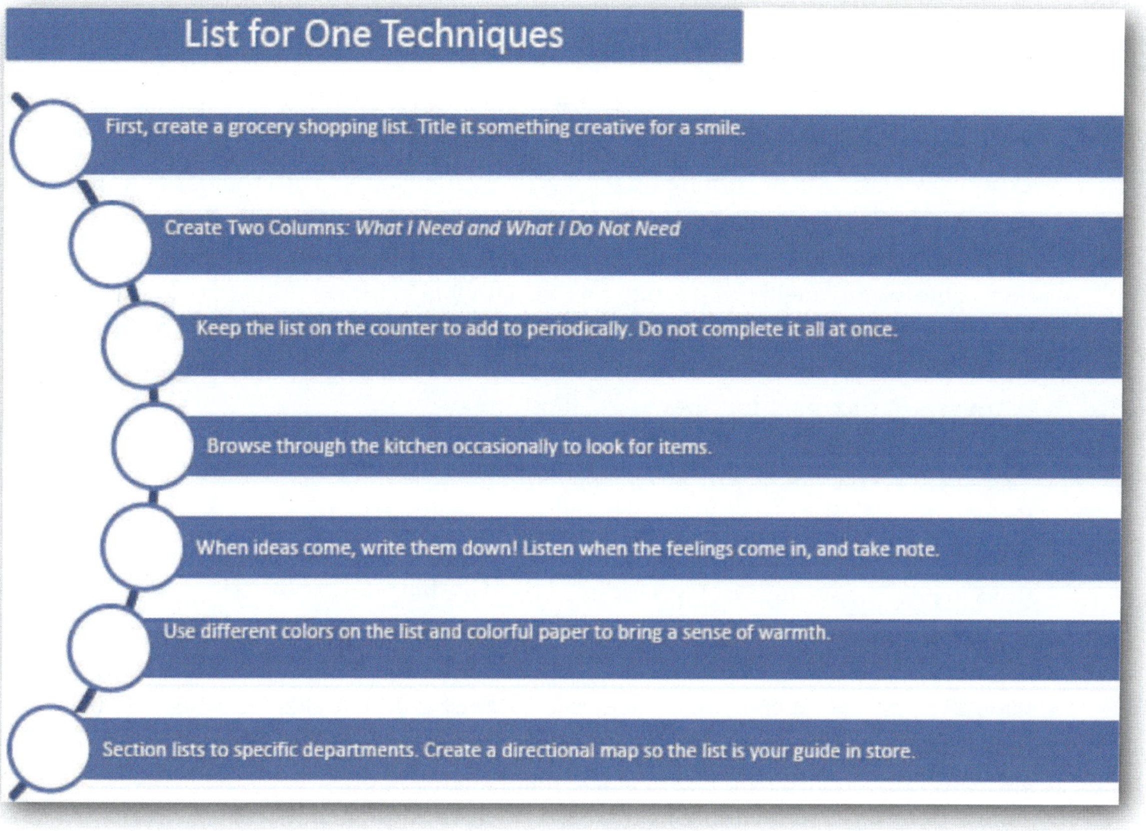

List-for-One Technique Descriptors

- *Create a Grocery List*
  The first task is to create a shopping list. Be sure to add a creative title rather than just calling it "Grocery List." It is important to begin the list with a sense of fun.

- *Create Two Columns: "What I Need" and "What I Do Not Need"*
  In creating your list, mark two separate columns on your sheet. Coming up with items can be difficult, especially at first. It can be intimidating to think of all the available items, let alone buying specific items just for one. Take a breath and prepare yourself. Your grocery list will look different now. This is one of the most difficult things to see on paper because your list will no longer include certain items you used to buy for your loved one. Take all the time needed to grieve this. Most often, the little things hit the hardest. The absence of certain items in your list is a significant factor, one that makes shopping for one truly difficult. On special holidays and occasions, think about

purchasing special items for remembrance and to feel the presence of the continuous bond shared with your loved one.

The two most important strategies in creating your list involve how you label each side and which side you complete first. First create a column titled "What I Do Not Need." Then create a column titled "What I Do Need"—in that order! This will alleviate the difficulty of trying to select grocery items. With that being said, if you begin to experience difficulty in coming up with grocery items, start with the basics. It is much easier to think of items you do not need than to select items that you do. Let's say you determine that you do not need lunch meat. Great! Once you put the item in the correct column, you are in the starting blocks. This will help you think of things you do in fact need. For example, lunch meat makes you think of tomato, lettuce, mustard, and so on. This serves as a grounding strategy and a reframing technique for the reduction of triggers in shopping-for-one.

- *Keep a List on the Counter to Periodically Add to*
  Keeping a list on the counter allows the grieving mind to "feel it as it comes." The grieving process is very complex, and this complexity makes it difficult to cognitively attend to tasks in just one sitting. Placing a list in a safe place helps ease the transition and reduce overwhelming emotions. Allow the brain to assess retrieval cues to certain stimuli. For example, if you see a commercial or smell a scent that induces a positive response or you notice someone enjoying a treat, take note of it in that exact moment. Otherwise the moment will pass, and the memory will be gone when you sit down later to create your list. Forgetfulness is one of the main cognitive grief responses. Therefore, you should purchase a small notepad and carry it with you at all times to help work through this symptom of grief. The act of writing or journaling as a means to making progress applies to all facets of grief, not just a grocery list. As mentioned in step two, journaling is a beautiful enrichment to the soul. It provides a psychosocial release of emotions in addition to normalizing and adjusting to multiple psychosocial grief responses. If we compare grief to an illness, journaling serves as an antibiotic. Just as you need to take all of your antibiotics, you need to stay consistent in the journaling. Even if you start to feel better, you do not stop taking your prescribed antibiotics—or writing, in this case.

- *Browse through the Kitchen Periodically to Look for Items*
  Browsing is an additional therapeutic method to assist with retrieval cues. Enter the kitchen calmly, and explore the cabinets, drawers, and refrigerator. Allow yourself to notice your reactions. If a specific item speaks to you, write it down. If nothing speaks to you, walk away. You do not want to force a reaction. The act of exposing yourself to the kitchen helps reduce triggers and heighted emotional responses in cooking-for-one. Continued exposure to the kitchen over time creates a positive emotional response in the long term. Therefore, take the time to become familiar with your kitchen again! Introduce your kitchen to the person you are now.

- *When Ideas Come, Write Them Down*
  Allow thoughts and feelings to come in without any judgment. As mentioned above, a very common cognitive grieving response is forgetfulness. Therefore, it is essential to write all ideas down as they arise. Otherwise, most thoughts will be forgotten. Additionally, in terms of writing, you want to "write it as you feel it." Your goal is to develop positive associations to food and the grocery store in order to help recondition positive feelings.

  For example, as soon as you start to experience hunger, immediately write down the food you imagine. Hunger is a positive response, associated with personal enjoyment. If the moment passes, you will lose the positive response. But if you write it down in the moment, you will capture the positive response and claim it as yours. Consequently, the next time you look at that item on your list, it will take you back to that thought and remind you of the pleasant response you experienced both physically and emotionally. On the other hand, if you write it down at a different time, you will not achieve a preconditioned response. That means you will not experience a positive emotional or physical response to the shopping because one was never identified or established.

- *Use Different Colors*
  Strategic use of color is a simple but important concept. In order to reduce the nerves, fear, and anxiety that come with shopping and cooking-for-one, you need to create a positive association with your list. A simple way to accomplish this is to make the presentation of the list fun and attractive. A plain piece of white paper does not evoke a warm, positive feeling, so use a color that makes you feel safe and hopeful. You should try to elicit a sense of hope.

  Furthermore, consider using different-colored writing utensils on the list at different times. This will help you remember specific feelings you experienced with various items you captured and wrote down. You want to make each item stand out. Changing colors at various times helps differentiate dates and feelings. In grief, we experience waves of emotions. We must aim to identify those waves and recognize each one that washes to shore. This enriches the soul and sends positive responses to the mind and body. Over time, this develops into a conditioned response and allows you to approach food, cooking, and grocery shopping with less anxiety, fear, and sadness.

- *Section Your List by Specific Departments: Map It*
  In order to help settle those rushing waves of grief, it is best to create a plan first and then create a directional map of the grocery store. Having a plan and a map will help to keep you from being overwhelmed at the front of the store, frozen in place and unsure where to start. As you make your list, make sure to group your items in their specific aisles. This is another reason it is important to choose a grocery store you are familiar with. Remember, the anticipation is typically worse than the actual shopping

experience. By creating a list and marking sections on a map of the store beforehand, you are reducing anxiety and fear. Now you have a plan. You will not get stuck at the front; you will know exactly where you are starting and will continue to follow your course until you reach the finish line. This coping strategy is also useful when you return home. There is nothing more difficult than coming home to an empty house without your loved one there to greet you. It can feel like a stab to the heart. This almost always elicits a frozen state. Try to use this coping strategy in coming home by having a plan for what to do as soon as you walk through the door. Section your home off on your mental map with a task you will attend to as soon as you walk through the door so you know where you will be going and what you will be doing. Consider simple tasks that you can move straight to.

Terms to become familiar with are task-brain and grieving-brain. In task-brain mode, your brain is centered on activating the process you previously developed to route your course. Doing so allows the task-brain to come forward and prevents the grieving-brain from keeping you stuck. The grieving-brain, on the other hand, only sees emptiness, isolation, and triggers. Imagine wearing two different lenses. The task-brain lens focuses on the process and how to accomplish the process. The grieving-brain lens focuses on loss and despair; this keeps tasks from being accomplished because the intensity of the grief is heightened to such a level that starting a task causes too much pain.

If you allow the grieving-brain to take control, negative and painful feelings develop into avoidance of cooking and grocery shopping. However, creating a list and mapping a plan allows the complicated grieving responses to take a back seat for a moment in order for you accomplish a task. In time you will be able to reframe negative thought patterns ("I will never be able to shop or cook-for-one") to rational thought patterns ("I *will* be able to shop and cook-for-one, slowly, in a new way"), which will elicit a healthier behavioral response. Ultimately, the process of grouping your list and mapping the store helps you ground your mind, body, and spirit and reduces the intensity of grief so that you can discover new experiences. Once this is achieved, you will no longer need to sit down and map out each task because doing so will be a learned skill.

Example of Sectioning Lists to Specific Departments

SHOPPING LIST	
PRODUCE	DAIRY
1 head of garlic	shredded jack cheese
2 lemons	package crumbled feta
2 mixed root vegetables	small container plain yogurt
1 red pepper	eggs
2 cups baby spinach	
1 pint cherry tomatoes	
celery	
¼ fingerling potatoes	
2 red onions	
GROCERY	MEAT
olive oil	1 rotisserie chicken
can chopped green chilies	bacon
2 cans chicken stock	Italian sausage
1 can white beans	ham
1 can tomato puree	
1 small box couscous	
1 box orzo	
small jar kalamata olives	

Step Five: Activate Your Task-Brain, and Rest Your Grieving-Brain

For further discussion, is essential to understand the difference between your task-brain and your grieving-brain. More important is to put forth effort throughout the day to create moments that direct your focus to task-brain activities in order to provide a mental break from the grieving-brain.

Task-brain activities are exactly what they sound like—activities focused on a task. When you direct your thoughts to a certain task or activity, feelings develop and attach to the specific task at hand, and this elicits positive responses and behaviors. Task-brain activities provide moments of distraction from grief symptoms; they allow grieving responses to settle for a moment. When the brain is focused on a task, all its energy is invested in that task. But when the brain is focused on grief, all that energy is invested in the grief symptoms. As a result, feelings of isolation, tears, and avoidance develop quickly, and the intensity of grief greatly magnifies.

In the context of cooking-for-one and shopping-for-one, it is vital to create plans that cause you to devote full energy to the task-brain. Consider creating a list, mapping a grocery store, or writing out directions to a recipe. These tasks require energy. But if no task process is initiated, intrusive thoughts will control that energy. The brain that is more powerful always takes the wheel. Because grief symptoms are some of the most powerful experiences one can have, the grieving-brain will dominate whenever there is not an identified task initiated. The symptoms of grief are remarkably intense, and grief itself is a magnet for negativity. It will quickly cling as tightly as it can to the nearest controllable target—you.

Therefore, it is best to write down directions prior to cooking and to use directions throughout the process to prevent the magnet from grabbing hold of you and pulling you back to bed (or away from the kitchen). Make a best-faith effort to push yourself to invest in a task in order to overcome the pull of the magnet. This will help you experience feelings of accomplishment and arrive at emotional responses of enjoyment, hope, and relaxation.

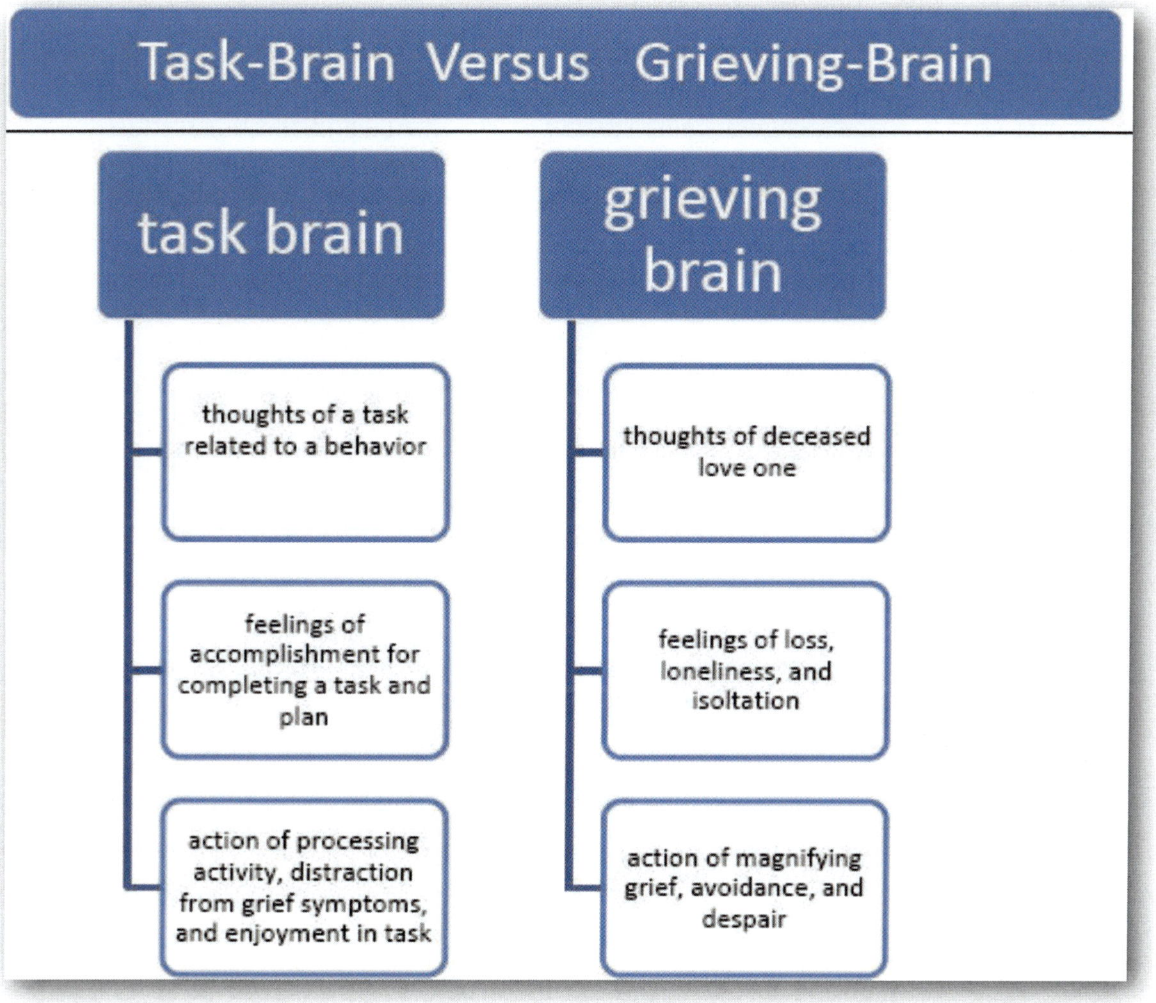
Task-Brain Versus Grieving-Brain
task brain
thoughts of a task related to a behavior
feelings of accomplishment for completing a task and plan
action of processing activity, distraction from grief symptoms, and enjoyment in task
grieving brain
thoughts of deceased love one
feelings of loss, loneliness, and isoltation
action of magnifying grief, avoidance, and despair

Step Six: Select Colors First

A very important step to take upon entering any grocery store is to select colors first. Your very first move in the store should be toward the colors. Colors affect emotion and behavior at a significant level. The psychology of color is based on the mental and emotional effects colors have on individuals who are grieving and in all facets of life. The goal with this step is to achieve a state of balance emotionally and physically to reduce the fears and anxieties that accompany cooking-for-one.

The act of moving toward colors upon entering the grocery store reduces the intensity of grief and fearful emotions. If at any point you are feeling overwhelmed, move toward the colors in the store. Allow yourself to mindfully observe the different colors around you. Notice all the colors and how they make you feel. This also serves as a distraction, as it utilizes the task-brain.

Most importantly, colors support healthy eating habits! The more color you add to your meals, the more nutrition you add to your diet. Many of the colorful food items at the grocery store have high nutritional values and are the best for you, such as blueberries, broccoli, corn, carrots, oranges, red peppers, tomatoes, and so on. Therefore, this step serves two purposes: it promotes healthy eating and relaxes the mind, body, and spirit so that you can comfortably shop-for-one.

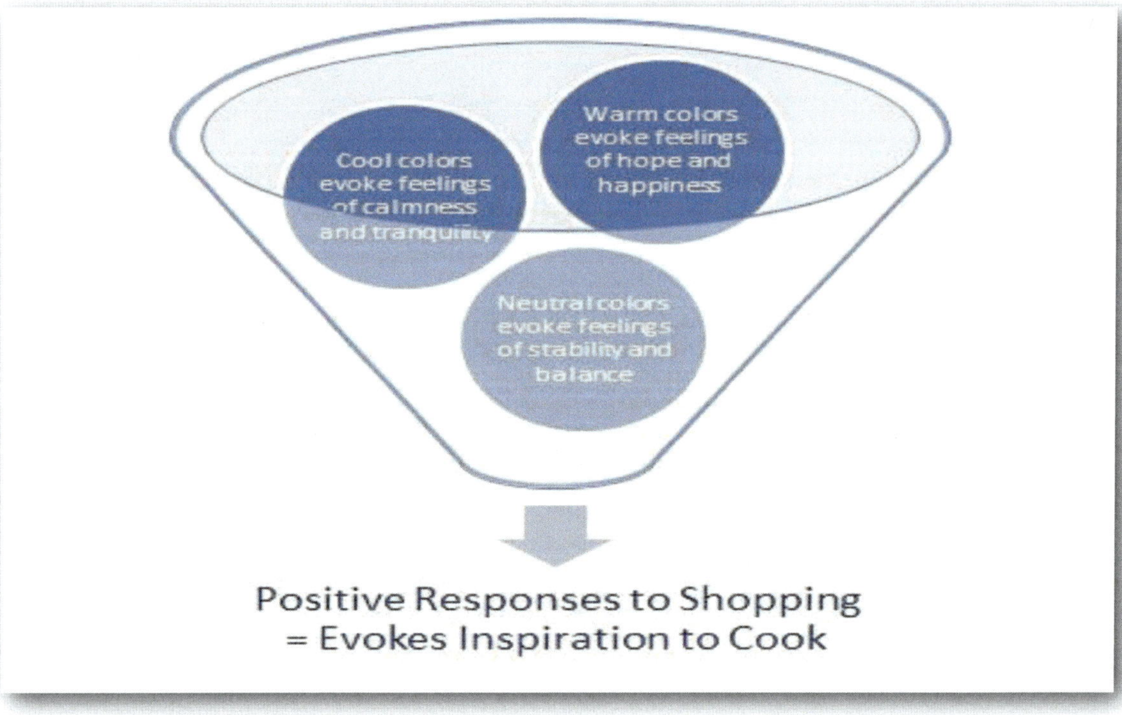

Step Seven: Ask for Help

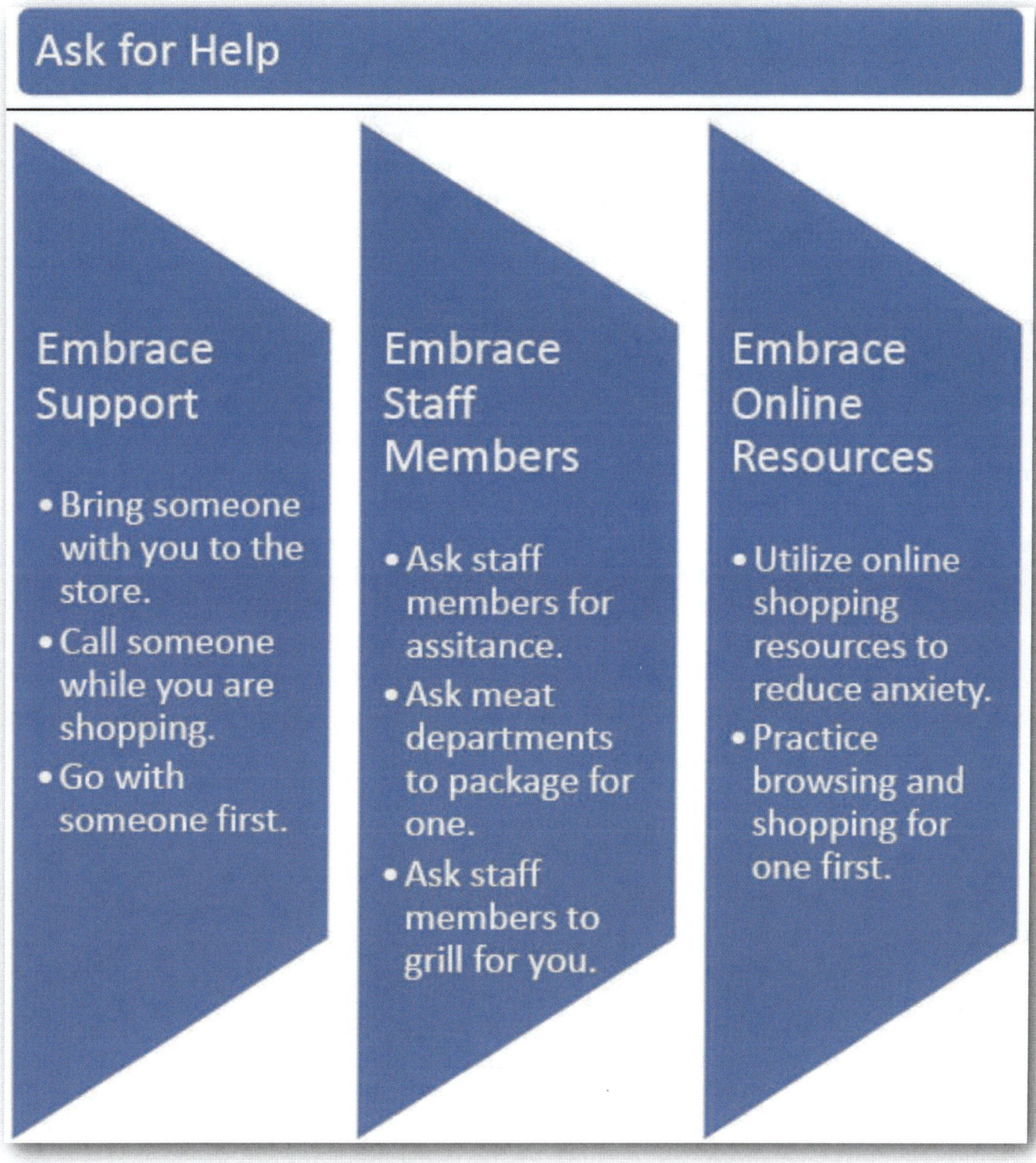

Refer to the Chart Above for Further Discussion:

Embrace Support

It is always best to tackle the grocery store with someone else first, whether it is to help with his or her shopping or to shop together. Consider who would be a safe person for this role.

Embrace Staff Members

Do not be timid about asking employees for help. If there is a food item you like but it is packaged in bulk, take it to the meat department and ask the butcher to repackage the item for one. Most employees are very happy to assist with this. In addition, consider grocery stores that have a grill on-site or provide seating for meals. Not only will the store grill the food item when you purchase it, but you can also eat it there. Many individuals eat at these sites by themselves, which is difficult to do at a formal restaurant. This provides an opportunity for exposure therapy: you can practice eating a meal out alone, a very difficult task after the loss of a loved one. Doing so at one of these locations, where you see more individuals than couples or families, can reduce the difficulty.

Embrace Online Resources

Ponder browsing and shopping for food online, especially if the grocery stores seem intimating or too difficult to tackle. If the cooking is more of a challenge for you, contemplate purchasing a meal service that is delivered to your own home. Not only does this eliminate the need to go to the store, but it also saves you from throwing away the leftovers. Several programs will deliver full-meal recipes (all the ingredients and directions) to your home; all you have to do is prepare the meal. This serves as a great motivator to continue practicing cooking-for-one, and it also lets you change up your routines to avoid becoming stagnant.

Step Eight: Use Grounding Exercises

Grounding exercises serve as anchors in the crashing waves of grief. They require the use of the senses to create a mind-body connection in the present.

Explore various grounding exercises until you find ones that feel most comfortable for you. You will want to practice utilizing these daily. Grounding exercises provide a sense of balance when flashbacks appear. For example, when you see couples at the grocery store, it may become difficult for you to catch your breath, and you may decide to leave. Using a grounding exercise will keep you at the store so that you can successfully complete your shopping trip.

Grounding exercises are not emergency care! Make sure to practice these exercises frequently—not just when you are stressed or upset, but also when you are relaxed. These exercises should become a habit of self-care to reflect healthy coping strategies.

Grounding Exercises

- Remind yourself who you are now. Say where you are now.
- Take five to ten deep breaths, and focus on each breath on the way in and the way out.
- Drink water.
- Utilize self-reflection or prayer.
- Squeeze a stress ball slowly and quickly, manipulating your breath with each squeeze.
- Examine the room, notice familiar objects, and name them. Notice any sounds and temperatures.
- Take a moment to notice your body. Notice any aches or pains. Notice any areas of warmth or coldness.
- Sit and feel the furniture you are resting upon. Are you supporting the chair, or is the chair is supporting you?
- Stop and listen. Notice and name what you can hear nearby and in the distance.
- Take a walk. Notice the feeling of each foot with every step.
- Sit outside, and notice the temperature of the air.
- Manipulate a fidget figure, which is a tactile tool manipulated with your hands, such as a stress ball, sliding cubes, therapy putty, tangle therapy, or texture tangibles to become engaged with a task.

Step Nine: Learn Proportioning and Sizing

It is difficult to determine sizing at a store off the top of your head. Consider using your own hand to help with quick measurements to break down recipes for one.

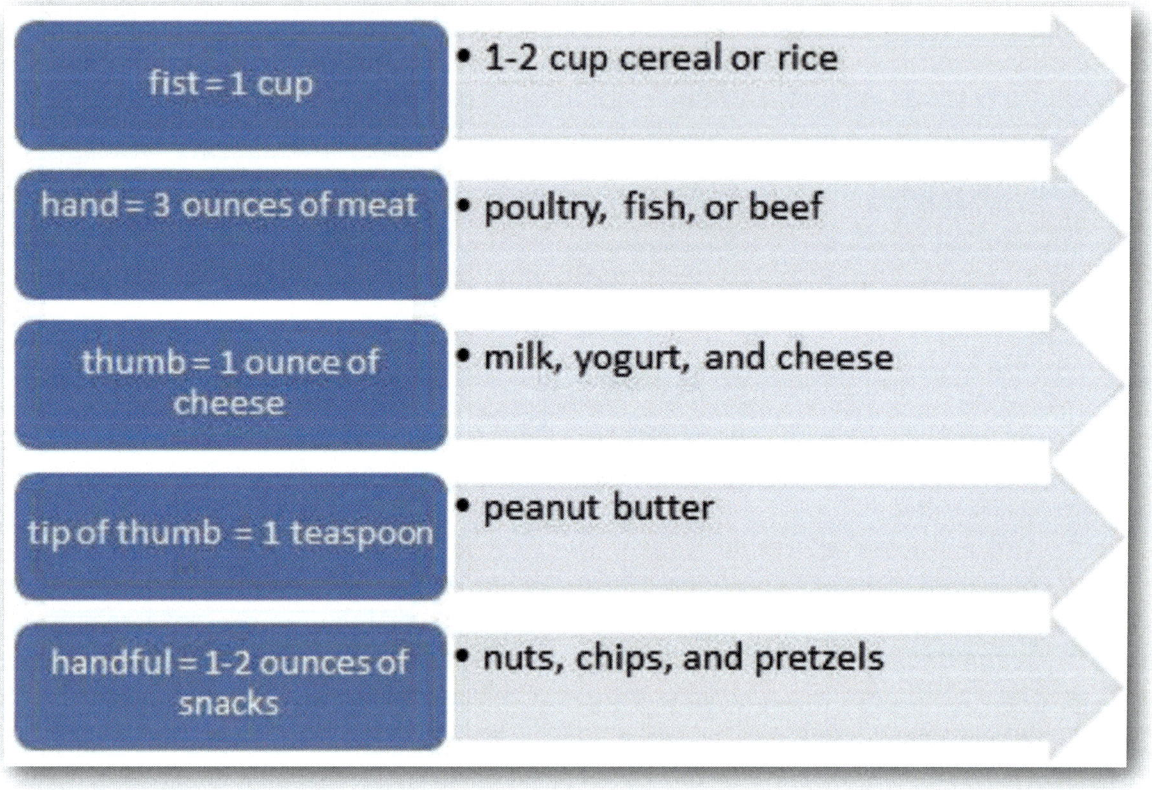

Step Ten: Reward Yourself

A significant step in grief work is rewarding yourself for your accomplishments. As mentioned above, in grief it is very common to focus solely on the steps still ahead. In doing so, we miss the opportunity to look back and see how far we have already come. We miss the opportunity to recognize our accomplishments.

In order to get to where you are going, you need to look back and see how you got to where you are today. Otherwise you may remain lost. It is essential to reward yourself for tasks completed and steps taken, even if they seem small to you. Grief work is about baby steps. Those baby steps are the pathway to the bigger steps of the journey.

Additionally, the act of rewarding yourself along the way creates positive associations with grocery shopping and cooking. An easy way to reward yourself is to pick up a special treat at the grocery store—something that was not on your original list. You can also stop for an ice cream on the way home or go someplace special to grab a bite to eat. Another option is to purchase something special for yourself that you have been waiting for. Take some time to consider what the best reward is for you, and change it up periodically to maintain the excitement factor. You want to avoid becoming stagnant or bored. We all need motivating factors to accomplish difficult tasks, and taking the time to recognize and reward our own strengths can provide that motivation.

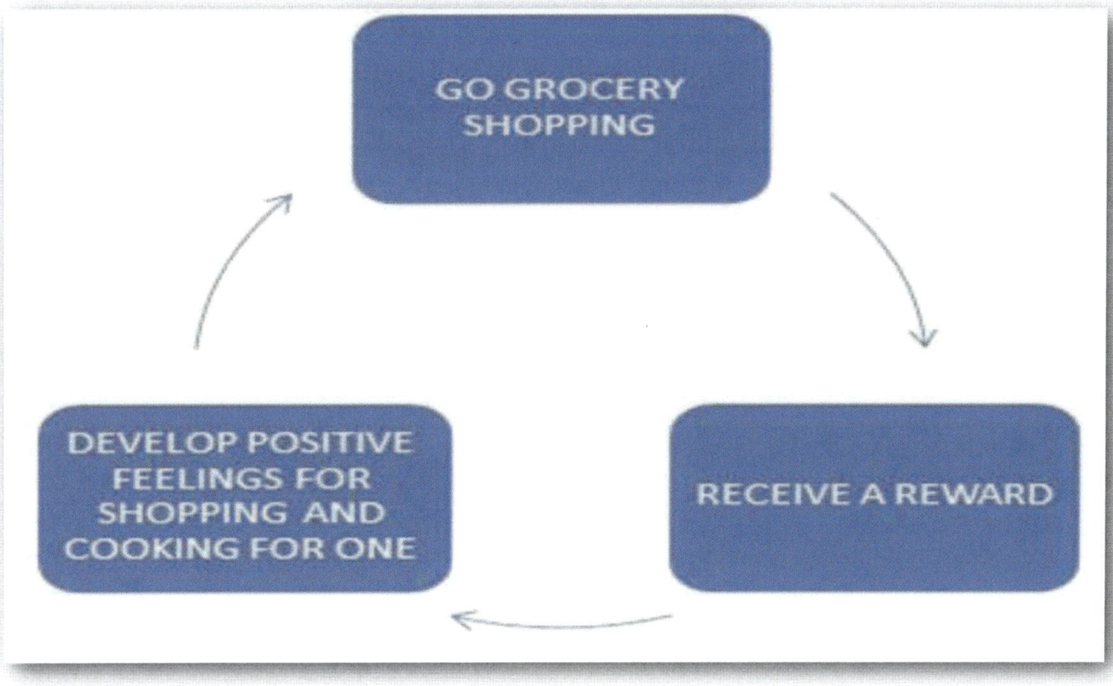

CHAPTER 2

Coping Techniques for Cooking-for-One

Change Routines

An essential coping technique in processing grief is to frequently change up your routines regarding cooking and mealtimes. You do not need to make drastic changes, just simple ones. The key is frequency, not severity.

Consider having your meals at a different time of day. For example, if you always had toast and coffee at 7:30 a.m., change the time to 8:30 a.m. Additionally, consider serving foods you typically did not have. For example, you might try Mexican or Chinese. Make an effort to experience different styles of food and different places to reduce triggers, create new schemas, and develop new associations.

Do not feel that you need to enjoy everything you try or that you always have to try new places. The key is to simply try. Your goal in engaging in new experiences is to eliminate triggers. By changing your routines at mealtimes, you will reduce painful triggers and flashbacks. In grief, the brain is very powerful; it fires off waves of emotions when you are engaged in familiar settings. Therefore, if you make an effort to remove the trigger, you will reduce the intensity of the associated pain response.

Further, consider changing the setting at mealtimes. Make an effort to assess all rooms, and choose the one that feels the least distressing. For instance, if the dining table brings you too much pain, eat in the living room or family room. Also, do not eat in silence. Put on the television or the radio to fill the room with sound. In grief, silence can be your worst enemy because it enables the mind to swirl in a whirlwind of emotions. Background noise reduces intrusive thoughts.

Another tip to consider is having meals outside occasionally. A breath of fresh air goes a long way toward grief reduction. First of all, eating outside is a grounding exercise in itself, as well as a mind and body enricher. Eating meals outside provides a positive setting in which to practice mindfulness exercises. While you are eating outside, take in all the elements around you. Listen to the birds singing hello to you, watch the squirrels running up the trees, and feel the sun or wind against your body, awakening your spirit and sending you signals of warmth and peace. Focusing on the elements of nature allows your heighted grieving responses to settle. Additionally, it eliminates exposure to the triggers inside the house. The physical act of stepping outdoors sends a message to the brain to strive for tranquility, even if only for a brief moment. Baby steps, remember?

The Rules of Weeknight Cooking-for-One

Rule One: Scale Down Recipes

Unfortunately, the recipe world is not designed for those who are grieving. Most recipes are written to feed at least four people. Therefore it is important to look for recipes that can be reduced to one or two portions. The Internet is a great resource for this because many online sites offer recipe converters and tips on how to scale a recipe back. While examining recipes, you should avoid bulky recipes unless you plan to freeze portions or share with others.

Example of Scaling Down a Recipe from Two to One

For Two	For One
1½ cups uncooked whole-grain pasta	¾ cups uncooked whole-grain pasta
1 cup asparagus, cut into 1-inch pieces	½ cup asparagus, cut into 1-inch pieces
6 ounces boneless, skinless chicken breasts, cubed	3 ounces boneless, skinless chicken breasts, cubed
2 cloves garlic, minced	1 clove garlic, minced
1 can (14½ ounces) diced tomatoes with juice	½ can (14½ ounces) diced tomatoes with juice
2 teaspoons dried basil or oregano	1 teaspoon dried basil or oregano
1 ounce soft goat cheese, crumbled	½ ounce soft goat cheese, crumbled
1 tablespoon Parmesan cheese	½ tablespoon Parmesan cheese

Rule Two: Keep It Simple

Weeknight cooking needs to be simple. More importantly, weeknight cooking-for-one needs to be extra simple. For starters, cooking-for-one means cleaning-for-one, so the more dishes you use while cooking, the more time you will spend cleaning. Consider using paper plates to avoid additional cleaning. It is essential to reduce the stress of cooking as much as possible, so avoid causing additional work for yourself. Your goal here is twofold: to feel a sense of accomplishment at the end and to eliminate feelings of exhaustion or stress. Although cooking for one takes effort and time, try to make all mealtimes positive experiences; such positive associations will encourage you to increase the frequency of your efforts.

Recipe for Keeping It Simple

Cha Cha's White Chicken Chili
2 servings

½ tablespoon vegetable oil
½ onion, chopped
1 clove garlic, crushed
½ can (2 ounces) chopped green chili peppers
1 teaspoon ground cumin
½ teaspoon dried oregano
½ teaspoon ground cayenne pepper
1 can (14½ ounces) chicken broth
1½ cups cooked chicken breast, chopped
1½ cans (22½ ounces) white beans
½ cup shredded Monterey Jack cheese (optional)

1. Heat the oil in a large saucepan over medium-low heat. Slowly cook and stir the onion until tender. Mix in the garlic, chili peppers, cumin, oregano, and cayenne. Continue to cook and stir the mixture until tender, about three minutes. Mix in the chicken broth, chicken, and white beans. Simmer fifteen minutes, stirring occasionally.
2. Remove the mixture from heat. Slowly stir in the cheese until melted. Serve warm.

Rule Three: Use Quick Cooking

Use the concept of quick cooking—do not set yourself up for an unattainable goal. Avoid using recipes that include a long list of ingredients and call for several cooking steps. When you start cooking-for-one, you need to be kind to yourself and create a positive atmosphere. Focus on items that can be prepared quickly, such as proteins and vegetables. Keep it simple: less is much more in this case.

Recipe for Quick Cooking

Avocado Strawberry Salad

3 cups arugula or mixed greens
½ pint strawberries, sliced
1 avocado, diced
2 ounces crumbled blue cheese
2 tablespoons sliced almonds, toasted
Sliced red onion to taste

½ cup cooked chicken breast, diced or pulled
Your favorite bottled poppy seed dressing

Place all ingredients in a large bowl. Toss with dressing to taste.

Rule Four: Soup Is Your Shadow

This next rule is the one exception to the big-batch rule. Soup can be portioned easily, and it freezes beautifully. It is a great option for the nights you just cannot find the strength to cook-for-one but you still want a healthy option. Soup can serve as your backup plan so that you can stay consistent with your cooking, as it provides the break you need when your grief is too heighted or intense for you to face your kitchen. Remind yourself that you are only human. Let soup be your shadow—always with you, especially when you need it the most.

Soup Recipe

Leftover Chicken Soup

1 chicken carcass (homemade or left over from a grocery-store rotisserie bird)
Water or chicken broth to cover (about 6 to 8 cups)
Salt and pepper to taste
1 onion, diced
6 carrots, peeled and sliced into coins
3 stalks of celery, cleaned and sliced
½ teaspoon dill or thyme
2 bay leaves
½ cup cooked small pasta (or any leftover you may have)

1. Place the chicken carcass in a large pot along with the onion, 3 carrots, 1 stalk of celery, and herbs. Pour in enough water or stock to cover. Bring to a boil and simmer for 2 to 3 hours.
2. Strain the soup through a fine-mesh strainer into another pot. Pick off any meat left on the bones, and add it to the soup. Discard the solids left in the strainer.
3. Add the remaining carrots and celery to the soup. Bring to a boil, and simmer until veggies are tender.
4. Add the cooked noodles to the pot, and season to taste with salt and pepper.

Rule Five: Eat a Sandwich

Sandwiches are an ideal choice when you are cooking-for-one. Sandwiches are fast, easy to make for one, and do not require any dishes. Additionally, sandwiches are very convenient, as you can make a sandwich from literally anything in your refrigerator. You can use leftover roasted vegetables, lunch meat, leftover chicken, salmon, and so on. Sandwiches are another healthy alternative for the nights you cannot find the strength to cook-for-one but want to stay consistent in your goal.

Sandwich Recipe

Grown-Up BLT

Dressing
¼ cup plain Greek yogurt
½ tablespoon chopped oregano
1 small clove garlic, minced
Kosher salt and pepper to taste

4 slices bacon
1 tomato, sliced
½ avocado, sliced
Lettuce leaves
4 slices white sandwich bread, toasted

1. Combine the dressing ingredients in a small bowl. Season to taste with salt and pepper.
2. Divide the toppings between the two sandwiches, and layer to your liking.

Rule Six: The Freezer Is Your Best Friend

The freezer is your best friend. It will help you eat healthier, stay consistent with cooking-for-one, and fight those cravings for microwave meals. Fill up your freezer with frozen produce or frozen meats that can be prepared quickly and easily, such as portioned chicken strips or steaks. Keep in mind that cooked grains freeze beautifully, as do pizza crusts and breads. Take some time to explore which foods are your favorites to freeze, and make sure to a keep a list handy to remind you to purchase these items each time you are at the grocery store or online. That way, these items will always be there for you when you need them the most—just like a best friend.

Freezer Recipe

Mini Lasagna Cups
Yield: 12 servings

2 Italian sausages, cooked and crumbled
1½ cups part-skim ricotta cheese

1 teaspoon Italian seasoning blend (feel free to use dry basil or oregano instead)
½ teaspoon salt
2 cups low-fat shredded mozzarella cheese
1 package square wonton wrappers
1½ cups store-bought tomato sauce of your choosing
Freshly ground black pepper

1. Preheat oven to 375°F. Lightly oil a standard muffin tin or spray with nonstick spray.
2. Place a wonton wrapper into each cup, and let the corners come over the edges. Make sure the wrapper is pressed firmly into each cup.
3. Season the ricotta cheese with salt and pepper to taste.
4. Mix the cooked sausage with the tomato sauce.
5. Into each cup place a tablespoon of the ricotta, a tablespoon of the marinara with sausage, and a tablespoon of mozzarella. Repeat with at least one more layer, or until each cup is full.
6. Bake ten to twelve minutes, or until the cheese on top is melted, browned, and bubbling.

Rule Seven: Do Not Fear the Leftovers

A significant fear for many people who are grieving and cooking-for-one is the concept of throwing away the leftovers. However, leftovers allow for creativity and thus engage the task-brain. Your goal should be to use the leftovers to create different dishes rather than making the same dish multiple nights. For example, the roasted chicken you made for dinner might become a chicken salad, a soup, or chicken tacos. Further, chili from last night's dinner makes a great topping for baked potatoes. The best part of having leftovers is it gives you an opportunity to have fun! You can try putting together all sorts of meals. Do not become discouraged if a meal does not come out "perfect." The object is to rediscover fun, reinvent who you are, and find your loved one's spirit in the process. Allow the fun to take hold of you, and do not use any judgment. Remember, the best ideas always come from those who take the risk to try.

Recipe for the Leftovers

Leftover Pasta

1 ounce olive oil
½ cup onion, chopped
2 cloves garlic, chopped
1 red, green, or yellow pepper, chopped
½ cup tomato (pureed, crushed, diced, or whole chopped)
2 to 3 cups chicken broth
1 cup cooked beans (white, black, or pinto)

2 cups cooked chicken or turkey
2 cups baby spinach
Basil or cilantro as desired
Salt and pepper to taste

1. Cook onions and garlic in olive oil over medium heat.
2. Add pepper, and cook for two minutes.
3. Add tomato, and cook for three to four minutes.
4. Add chicken broth and beans. Simmer for ten to fifteen minutes.
5. Add chicken, spinach, and herbs. Simmer for five minutes.
6. Adjust seasoning.

You can also use all vegetables and vegetable broth for a vegetarian option.

Rule Eight: Do Not Be Afraid to Ask

Do not be afraid to ask the staff at the grocery store to repackage items, such as meat or fish, in smaller portions. You can bring any item to the meat market and ask the staff to repackage it for you. You do not only have to purchase an item directly from the meat market itself to do this. In most stores, the staff will repackage an item you purchased anywhere in the store. Do not be afraid to ask for help; you will find that many people request this.

Rule Nine: Plan Meals for the Week

Purchase a chicken or a pot roast. Yes, a chicken or a pot roast is a lot of food, not to mention a large time commitment, but you can use it over the course of a few days. It can also be turned into different dishes that can be frozen for later use. For example, a whole chicken becomes chicken wraps on Monday, chicken tacos on Tuesday, and a white-bean chicken chili on Wednesday. The only rule here is to make sure you do not create too much. You do not want to store meat in your fridge for more than three or four days. Therefore, if you plan to make a larger roast, be sure to purchase appropriate supplies to freeze the additional leftovers to avoid any setbacks or discouragements. It is best to plan your meals for the week by using the leftovers from the first day and creating different dishes for the following days. Doing so keeps you from throwing away extra food and spending more money, and it saves a great deal of time and energy. Grief itself is very exhausting and depletes energy. Planning for the week is a healthy coping strategy that helps to alleviate negative responses and symptoms by conserving your energy.

Recipes for Weekly Meal Planning

Herb-Roasted Chicken with a Mix of Roasted Root Vegetables
Herb-Roasted Chicken

1 (3½- to 4-pound) whole chicken
1½ tablespoons salt
2 teaspoons black pepper
1 tablespoon garlic, minced
1 tablespoon thyme leaves, chopped
½ tablespoon sage leaves, chopped
2 tablespoons parsley leaves, chopped (reserve the stems)
½ cup olive oil
1 lemon, quartered
2 bay leaves

Root Vegetables

¼ pound turnips, peeled and medium diced
¼ pound carrots, peeled and medium diced
¼ pound parsnips, peeled and medium diced
¼ pound golden beets, peeled and medium diced
¼ pound red beets, peeled and medium diced
¼ pound fingerling potatoes, halved
1½ teaspoons salt
½ teaspoon black pepper
¼ cup olive oil

1. Preheat the oven to 475°F.
2. Wash the chicken, and pat dry. Season well inside and out with the salt and pepper.
3. In a small bowl, combine the garlic, thyme, sage, parsley, and olive oil. Rub the olive oil blend into the cavity of the chicken as well as all over the exterior. Place the parsley stems into the cavity of the chicken. Squeeze each lemon quarter into the chicken, and place the rind in as well. Put the bay leaves inside the chicken, place the bird in a roasting pan or a sauté pan, and put it into the oven. Roast for about one hour, or until the chicken is golden brown and the juices run clear. Remove from the oven and let sit for ten minutes before carving.
4. Place the vegetables in a large mixing bowl, and season with the salt and pepper. Drizzle with the olive oil, and place in a roasting pan or on a sheet pan. Place in the oven and roast for thirty minutes, turning once midway during cooking to ensure even browning. Serve with the herb-roasted chicken.

Israeli Couscous with Roasted Vegetables

½ cup Israeli couscous (not Moroccan)
½ tablespoon fresh lime juice

½ teaspoons curry powder
¼ teaspoon cumin
⅛ teaspoon coriander
½ teaspoon pure chili powder
1 tablespoon extra-virgin olive oil
Leftover roasted root vegetables
2 teaspoons fresh cilantro, chopped
2 teaspoons fresh Italian (flat-leaf) parsley, chopped
Kosher salt and freshly ground black pepper to taste

1. Boil one quart of water with a pinch of salt. Add couscous to boiling water, and cook according to directions. Drain couscous, and toss with half the olive oil. Spread onto a flat pan to cool.
2. Mix together in a bowl the remaining olive oil, lime juice, curry, cumin, coriander, chili powder, cilantro, and parsley.
3. Gently toss couscous, vegetables, and vinaigrette in a large bowl. Adjust seasoning with salt, pepper, or more spices. Let marinate one hour before serving.

Chicken Salad

1 cup chopped chicken (from leftover roasted bird)
¼ cup mayonnaise or more to taste
1 tablespoon lemon juice
Salt and pepper to taste
1 stalk celery, chopped
Optional: grapes, almonds, blue cheese, fresh herbs, red onions

Place all ingredients in small bowl, and mix to combine.

Rule Ten: Find Joy in Cooking-for-One

First of all, step outside of your own head when it comes to what *fun* means. Fun, in this context, means playing music in the background, having an enjoyable show on, or talking to a loved one on the phone. This way, you can enjoy the music, television show, or company of a good friend while cooking to help use task-brain instead of grieving-brain. Allow the music, the show, or the friend to distract you and ease your mind. The act of directing your focus to these tasks engages your task-brain and puts you in control of your thought patterns. This creates a more positive cooking experience and reduces intrusive or negative thoughts.

Fun also means using colorful paper plates to avoid doing the dishes. Make it a point to pick fun colors. Of course, if you want to break out the fine china, please do so!

Remember, you have a great number of accomplishments to be proud of (even if it does not seem like it). Make sure to recognize your resilience because it is present in every action you take. It is present when you push yourself to get out of bed every day and continue to climb a mountain of grief, step after step, even though it is so hard to see the peak. Unfortunately, some individuals do not understand how heavy one step can be and how much effort you put forth in that one step, just to do it all over with a new one. However, we do. And you need to see that, too. Give yourself permission to find a little joy in cooking—you owe it to yourself and your loved one. Let your loved one's spirit come alive through the art of cooking, and use your senses to guide you closer to him or her. You can truly experience that back-in-time feeling through cooking and thus build a stronger continuous bond. Do not let the fear of trying to cook-for-one keep you from reaching your loved one in a way that is possible now. Use the culinary arts as your flashlight in the dark mist of grief. Cooking will guide you to the path of integration, which is discovering a new sense of meaning, purpose, and happiness through the heart of your loved one.

CHAPTER 3

Cooking-for-One Recipes for Different Themes and Seasons

Cooking-for-one is a difficult process to master. Therefore, it is essential to have multiple go-to recipes in times of need.

Consider creating a recipe book for your journey. This way, the recipes will be easily accessible, and you can refer back to them at any time. The book itself encourages accountability, making it easier to stay consistent with your grief-therapy goals.

The recipes listed below pertain to specific grieving stages, days, and themes that are most difficult. The purpose of these special recipes is to serve as support and motivation through the difficult days and the gotchas to reduce the likelihood of the quick fix—grabbing junk food or microwave meals.

Consider creating your own titles for certain days or specific triggers pertinent to you, and add recipes that are fitting to you. Doing so will generate a greater response because it will mean more to you and provide a road map for your journey. Take time to explore what your difficult days and gotchas are. Of course, you will not be able to record all of them, as grief happens in unpredictable and unanticipated waves, but you can record those that are known to you. Once you've done that, record a recipe that elicits a healthy response and inspires support, hope, and comfort.

Recipe for the Days You Cannot Get Out of Bed or Stop the Tears

There are days when the intensity of grief is so strong that it seems as if your ankles are anchored down to the bed. On these days, it is important to have something to find comfort in to swim against the crashing waves. Consider a warm meal to help provide a hug and keep you on your feet to fight the pull back to bed.

Bacon Macaroni and Cheese

8 ounces elbow macaroni
1 can condensed cheddar cheese soup
1 cup milk
3 cups shredded sharp cheddar cheese (save 1 cup for topping)

1½ tablespoons butter, melted
8 ounces bacon, cooked and crumbled
Salt and pepper to taste

1. Preheat oven to 350°F. Grease a 9 × 13 baking dish and set aside.
2. Cook pasta according to package directions. Drain and put back in pot with remaining ingredients, and mix well.
3. Pour into baking dish, sprinkle with reserved cup of cheddar, and bake until top is golden brown and bubbly.

Recipe for Eating Outdoors to Catch Some Fresh Air

It is very important to change the scenery in order to reduce conditioned grief trigger responses. Consider having a meal outdoors on the days you need to catch your breath. This will help you to relax and practice mindfulness. Think of this recipe on the days you feel the walls closing in.

2 wedge bratwurst links
1 large unpeeled Granny Smith apple
¼ small red onion
2 tablespoons mayonnaise
1 teaspoon cider vinegar
½ teaspoon spicy brown mustard
⅛ teaspoon celery salt
2 hoagie rolls

1. Preheat grill to medium-high. Grill brats until cooked through, turning often, about ten to twelve minutes.
2. Grate apple and red onion into large bowl. Toss with mayo, vinegar, mustard, and celery salt.
3. Place brats on hoagie rolls, and top with slaw.

Recipe for Lifting Your Spirits

Everyone who is grieving needs a little motivation and an extra push, as the journey is truly exhausting. Reflect on this recipe on the days you need an extra boost of inspiration. Give yourself permission to climb and reach heights you feel are impossible to achieve. You will surprise yourself with the strength you have if you just give yourself the chance to see it. Make sure to take time to reflect on your power and enjoy your victory meal.

Pasta with Vodka Sauce and Sausage

¼ pound pasta
1 tablespoon olive oil
¼ pound Italian sausage, removed from the casing and crumbled or chopped
½ cup yellow onions, chopped
½ teaspoon salt
Pinch crushed red pepper flakes
2 teaspoons garlic, minced
½ cup crushed tomatoes
3 tablespoons vodka
2 tablespoons heavy cream
1 to 2 tablespoons fresh basil, chopped
Parmesan cheese for topping

1. Bring a medium saucepan of salted water to a boil. Add pasta, and cook until done. Drain and return to the saucepan.
2. While the water boils and the pasta cooks, heat the olive oil in a skillet over medium heat. Add the sausage and cook, breaking up the meat until browned (no pink left). Add the onions, salt, and red pepper flakes, and cook until the onions are soft and begin to turn golden. Add the garlic and tomatoes, and cook, stirring, until thick, about two minutes. Add the vodka, and cook until the sauce is reduced by half. Stir in the cream, and cook until the sauce thickens. Stir in the basil, and remove from the heat.
3. Toss the sauce with the pasta to coat evenly, and transfer to a pasta bowl for serving. Top with cheese if desired.

Recipe for the Good Days

We all experience good days and bad days. Even on the good days, we need to find the fuel to keep us running strong. Practice using recipes that inspire hope and keep motivation present. Think of this recipe as a pit stop at the gas station to fill up.

Grapefruit and Avocado Salad

1 tablespoon cider vinegar
1 tablespoon honey
2 tablespoons Dijon mustard
3 tablespoon olive oil
Salt and pepper to taste

¼ red onion, chopped
¼ cup feta cheese, crumbled
4 tablespoons sesame seeds
¾ pound baby spinach
1 grapefruit, peeled with sections cut free from membranes

1. Whisk the vinegar, honey, mustard, and olive oil together to make dressing.
2. In a large serving bowl, mix remaining ingredients with about half of the dressing, and adjust seasoning to taste.

Recipe for Grieving during the Holidays

For the first year of loss, consider a holiday meal different from what you typically serve. Switch up the food in regard to what you cook, or even have the meal catered. It is important to remember that what you do the first year is not what you have to do the next. For the second year of loss, contemplate having a meal your loved one truly enjoyed, and share a special dish in honor of him or her. Or perhaps recognize a dish your loved one always wanted to have. For all years, take into account sharing with family and friends how your loved one was a gift to you. Ask family members to write down something that tells how your loved one was a gift. You can share how your loved one made you feel, ways he or she made you laugh, things he or she did to support you, something you learned from him or her, and so on. Children can also draw pictures to express their thoughts. Once all of you have finished writing, place your piece of paper into a gift box or a memory box. Then, before enjoying the meal or opening the gifts, think over reading these out loud as a remembrance of the greatest gift in life itself—your loved one.

Spinach-Artichoke Dip

2 cups Parmesan cheese
1 box (10 ounces) frozen chopped spinach, thawed and drained of excess liquid
1 can (14 ounces) artichoke hearts, drained and chopped
⅔ cup sour cream
1 cup cream cheese
⅓ cup mayonnaise
2 teaspoons garlic, minced

1. Preheat oven to 375°F.
2. Mix together Parmesan cheese, spinach, and artichoke hearts.
3. Combine remaining ingredients, and mix with spinach mixture.
4. Bake for twenty to thirty minutes.
5. Serve with crackers or toasted bread.

Recipe for the Fall

Each season sets the stage for a new milepost on your journey, almost like a checkpoint in a marathon. Consider having recipes to use as checkpoints to mark a sense of accomplishment and motivate you to reach the goals ahead. Look at setting a cooking goal for a certain time frame each week, every other week, or every month. Set a realistic goal you know you will accomplish. Ultimately, it is more productive to obtain a goal versus setting a goal too high to reach.

Butternut Squash Bisque

1 package (20 ounces) precut butternut squash
½ red pepper, roughly chopped
½ medium yellow onion, roughly chopped
1 clove garlic, smashed and peeled
3½ cups water
½ tablespoon salt
1 tablespoon sugar
¼ cup heavy cream
Fresh thyme sprigs for garnish

1. In a large pan, combine everything but the cream and thyme sprigs. Bring it to a boil, cover, and simmer until the vegetables are very soft.
2. Puree the soup until smooth. You may do this in the pan with an immersion blender or in batches in a blender.
3. Return the soup to the pan (if necessary), and stir in the heavy cream. Bring the soup to a simmer, but do not boil, as this may cause the cream to break.
4. Taste the soup, and adjust the seasonings to your liking. Garnish with chopped thyme.

Recipe for the Winter

Winter is one of the most difficult seasons for those who are grieving because the nights bleed into the days. Likewise it is one of the most difficult times to cook-for-one because the intensity of grief will be at its highest. It is important to have hobbies in the home and to stay consistent with stocking the fridge with food items. If you have the food items in your home, you will be more inclined to stay consistent in cooking because you will not want them to go to waste. Recognize that this season will be a challenge and keep a to-do list posted in clear view to help you stay accountable. Also practice setting a reminder or a timer on your phone to remind you to go to the grocery store. It is vital to set reminders because the person who may have served as your reminder is not able to do so anymore. When there's no one to nudge you, it is easy to put off these tasks. When you create reminders, consider using the language or phrases your loved one used to use. You know what he or she would say; let yourself hear it again.

Root Vegetable Hash with Egg

½ pound beets, peeled and diced
¼ yellow onion, chopped
2 ounces sweet potatoes, peeled and diced
6 ounces Yukon Gold or white boiling potatoes, peeled and diced
1 tablespoon olive oil
1 garlic clove, minced
1 tablespoon fresh flat-leaf parsley, chopped
1 egg, fried or poached
Salt and pepper to taste

1. Preheat oven to 400°F.
2. Pour the olive oil into a baking pan large enough to hold the vegetables in a single layer. Add the vegetables, and sprinkle with the garlic and the salt and pepper. Roast, stirring every fifteen minutes to scrape up the browned bits, until vegetables are tender, about forty-five to fifty minutes. Stir in the parsley.
3. Place the hash on a plate, and wash with an egg. Season with salt and pepper, and serve immediately.

Recipe for the Spring

The weather is starting to get warmer, and the days are starting to get longer, which means it is a perfect time to start adding more inspiration into your recipes. Use the extra daylight to help you get to the store and lift your mood to cook more. Recognize recipes that help fulfill the daylight.

Chopped Salad

2 cups cooked ditalini pasta
1½ cups romaine lettuce, chopped
1½ cups iceberg lettuce, chopped
1 cup red cabbage, chopped
1 fresh tomato, diced
½ cup green onions, diced
½ cup bacon, cooked and crumbled (or real bacon bits)
2 ounces Gorgonzola cheese (you could add up to 8 ounces if you *really* like Gorgonzola)
1 cup chicken, cooked and diced (optional)
Your favorite bottled balsamic vinaigrette

1. Cook pasta according to instructions. Drain in a colander, rinse with cool water, and set aside.

2. Combine romaine, iceberg, red cabbage, tomatoes, and green onions in large salad bowl.
3. Add cooled pasta, bacon, and Gorgonzola cheese to salad. Add dressing to taste before serving.

Recipe for the Summer

Summer is the season of the longest daylight. Take advantage of the longer days by switching up mealtimes. Consider having meals earlier or later, and explore meals in different settings. Ponder having a meal at a park instead of your backyard. At a park, there are typically several people eating alone, which helps reduce the isolation factor or the spotlight feeling of eating-for-one. This is an ideal time to practice eating-for-one. See about barbequing-for-one, since this is a great way to avoid wasting leftovers. Grilling meals is a great way to minimize leftovers. For example, it is simple to grill up chicken breasts for one meal and then turn the leftovers into a chicken salad the next day and a chicken wrap the following day. The grill is great tool for creating multiple meals from leftovers and practicing weekly meal planning.

Pork Kebabs with Lemon Rice

1 pound pork tenderloin
6 tablespoons lemon juice
Zest from 1 lemon
4 tablespoons olive oil
3 cloves of garlic, minced
1½ tablespoons oregano
1½ teaspoons kosher salt, divided
½ teaspoon freshly ground black pepper
½ cup white rice
½ tablespoon butter
1 tablespoon Italian parsley, minced

1. Trim any silver skin or fat off the pork, and cut into 1-inch chunks. Place in a bowl.
2. In a separate bowl, mix the olive oil with 4 tablespoons of the lemon juice, the garlic, oregano, salt, and black pepper. Pour over the pork, and mix to combine. Cover with plastic wrap and marinate, refrigerated, for at least 2 hours.
3. Heat grill to medium-high heat. Remove the pork from the marinade, and discard the marinade. Thread the meat on metal or wooden skewers. If using wooden skewers, make sure to soak them in water for at least 30 minutes before using.
4. In a small saucepan combine 1 cup of water, the rice, lemon zest, reserved lemon juice, butter, and 1 teaspoon of salt. Bring the rice to a boil. Cover, reduce heat to low, and simmer for 20 minutes. Let the rice rest for at least 5 minutes. Fluff with a fork, and adjust seasoning if necessary.

5. Grill the pork until browned and cooked to your desired level of doneness (about 7 to 10 minutes). Remove to a platter, and serve with lemon rice.

Recipe for Birthdays

Use this recipe or a food or drink recipe that your loved one specifically enjoyed. Practice journaling as you enjoy this recipe, and write to your loved one about everything you want to share with him or her at this yearly milestone.

Portillo's Style Chocolate Cake

1 Betty Crocker Super Moist Favorites Butter Recipe Chocolate Cake Mix
3 large eggs
1 cup water
1 cup Hellmann's mayonnaise (not light)

1. Preheat oven to 350°F.
2. Grease two round cake pans (or your choice of pan; cupcakes work great too).
3. Beat all ingredients for four minutes (until fluffy).
4. Pour into prepared pans.
5. Follow baking instructions on box for your choice of pan, elevation, and the like.

Recipe to Reward Yourself and Recognize Your Strengths

Not only is it important to take the time to recognize your strengths, but it is also important to reward yourself for the milestones you have accomplished. Explore recipes that provide a sense of accomplishment and resilience. You are the true definition of resilience; let the recipes help you see that.

Boston Cream Icebox Cake

Cake
3 cups milk
1 package (16 ounces) graham crackers
1 container (8 ounces) Cool Whip
2 packets instant vanilla pudding

Topping
1 cup sugar
½ cup (1 stick) butter
½ cup semisweet chocolate, finely chopped or chips

¼ cup milk
1 teaspoon vanilla

1. Line a 9 × 13 pan with parchment paper or aluminum foil. Then cover completely with one layer of graham crackers, breaking the grahams into smaller pieces to fill gaps.
2. In a large bowl, combine pudding packets, Cool Whip, and milk, and pour half of the mixture evenly over grahams.
3. Add another layer of graham crackers, and top with remaining pudding mixture and one final layer of graham crackers.
4. For the topping, combine all ingredients in a saucepan over medium heat, stirring frequently.
5. Once chocolate, butter, and sugar have melted completely and all ingredients are fully incorporated, remove from heat and pour evenly over top layer of graham crackers.
6. Cover tightly and freeze at least four hours, or overnight.

CHAPTER 4

Mindful Eating

Mindful eating is eating with intention and attention. When you are grieving, mindful eating helps you take care of yourself while enjoying a meal and reducing painful triggers. In order to accomplish this, start eating your meals with an intention to take care of yourself, such as recognizing the strength in the beautiful meal you prepared. Start eating with attention by noticing and enjoying your food and its effects on your body. This process involves your task-brain, which helps reduce intrusive thought patterns.

Become aware of any physical and emotional cues toward food. Notice how food makes you feel on both levels. In order to experience a reaction, be sure to choose foods for both enjoyment and nourishment. This way, you will experience a feeling of satisfaction and develop a healthier relationship with cooking and eating-for-one.

Your goal is to react mindfully and not mindlessly. If you react mindlessly, triggers, intrusive thoughts, and intense feelings rush in, which leaves you feeling powerless to change and powerless in taking steps to cook-for-one. Mindfulness increases your awareness of these patterns without judgment and creates a space between your triggers and your actions, providing an atmosphere where you can finally enjoy a meal and feel a sense of hope that cooking-for-one is possible. Mindful eating empowers a sense of peace, even at mealtimes.

To practice mindful eating, please refer to the diagrams below. The main objective is to utilize all of your senses while engaging in eating.

MINDFUL EATING TIPS

First, observe the food and notice all the aspects of color, shape, size.

Then, notice the smell of the food. How does it affect you? Does it remind you of any specific memories? Where, when, and why? Record these.

Continue to examine the taste of the food.

First, simply introduce the food to your mouth–do not take a whole bite.

Notice all initial reactions as the food hits your mouth. Do you feel any warmth or coolness? Let the taste remind you of memories in time. Record these.

Then, take a bite of the food–do not swallow in one mouthful. Notice how the food feels to chew and how it affects your body. Notice the memories.

Finally, swallow the food and notice how it feels in your throat and down to your stomach. Record the process.

Practice a mindful bite at the start of every meal upon cooking and eating-for-one. Afterward, continue to eat at your pleasure. Practicing a mindful bite at the start of all meals is also practicing relaxation, which reduces intrusive thoughts and grief triggers and leads to positive responses toward mealtimes and cooking-for-one. It is helpful to use self-reflection during this exercise by recording what memories come to mind as you smell and taste the food. Use those senses to help you recreate moments and elicit a "back in time" feeling. Write what comes to mind as you taste and smell the food. You can even take it a step further, writing what you want to say to your loved one.

CHAPTER 5

Incorporating Food with Tasks

In introducing the concept of cooking-for-one, it is helpful to incorporate food with certain tasks in order to associate cooking and mealtimes with a sense of joy and hope. If you are going to cook or eat a meal, make sure to combine it with a task to provide a bit of pleasure in the difficult grieving process.

CONSIDER SHARING YOUR MEALS WITH...

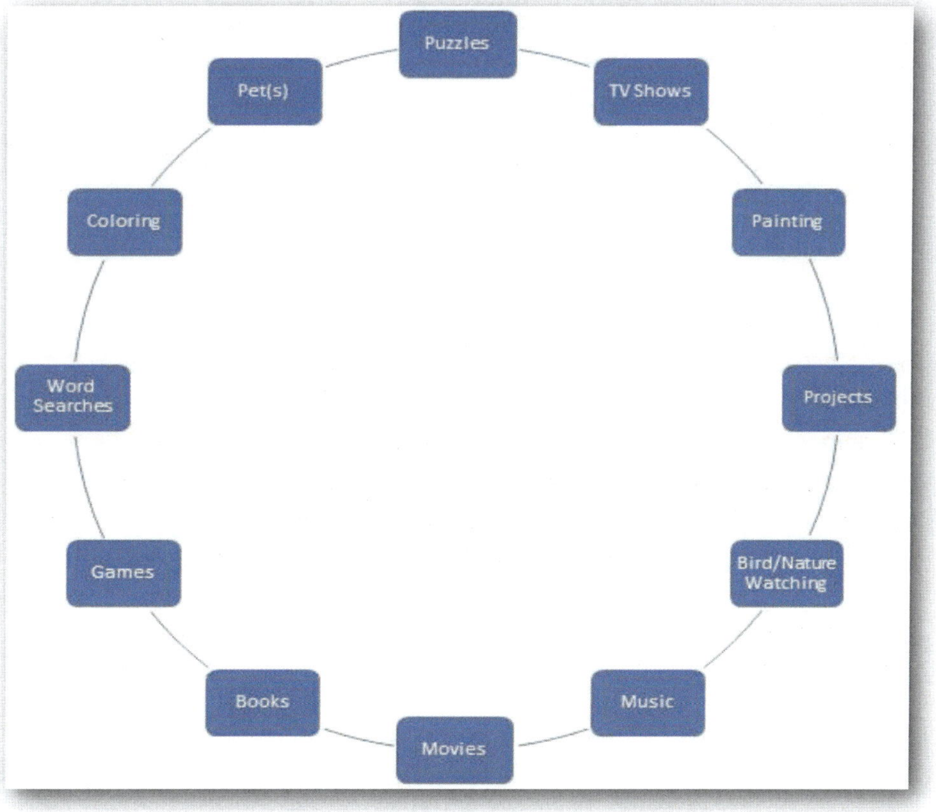

CHAPTER 6

Continuous Bonds—Celebrating Life with Food

Cooking is actually a beautiful way to honor your loved one, remain connected, and share his or her spirit and presence with other people. Food is a tangible measure to allow your loved one to live on.

Take a few moments to think about how many recipes are passed down from generation to generation and the stories behind those recipes. More importantly, think about the meaning, purpose, and value those recipes hold. For instance, a mother gives her son a recipe for his father's famous root beer floats. With that recipe she includes a note about how he would always have one of these on special occasions. The hope is that on special occasions in the son's life, he will have a root beer float and feel as if his dad is there with him. On the days we need our loved ones the most, we can find them through the culinary arts.

For special dates, holidays, and occasions, take note of certain meaningful recipes, and use them to connect with your loved one. You can find your loved one in the atmosphere of food and speak to him or her through your cooking.

For instance, if your spouse made the perfect vanilla milkshake, make sure to purchase those special ingredients and have a toast to him or her. While you enjoy your milkshake, talk to your spouse, saying everything you want him or her to know. Use those moments to represent life. You have all the power to bring a loved one's spirt and essence to life. Do not be afraid to go there. Yes, it will be difficult, but once you make it, you will be glad you did.

Our senses make grief tangible. Our senses show us pieces we cannot see. Our senses connect us to our loved one in a physical manner. Use the culinary arts to take you there. While you prepare a meal or a drink, put a loved one's favorite song on, and let it play loudly. Do not be afraid to cry. Your tears are memories you should wear proudly.

Find your loved one in the taste, sight, sound, touch, and, most importantly, the smell of the foods you prepare. The sense of smell is one of the strongest senses in grief work. Our sense of smell can unravel unlimited avenues of emotions, memories, and connections. Scents offer both psychological and physical benefits. Not only does the aroma of the food or drink stimulate the brain to trigger a positive reaction, but it also supplies therapeutic benefits when it is inhaled into the lungs.

Further, there is no filter with scents: a scent goes directly to the brain. Smells trigger vivid emotional memories and are stronger at inducing the feeling of being brought back in time than images or pictures. The sense of smell can truly recapture a scene and a period in time, which makes culinary grief therapy so important.

If you feel far away from your loved one, allow his or her scent to bring you back in time to those precious moments you need the most. A smell can truly conjure the person, more than just looking at a photo. You actually get the feeling of the person from the smell. Ultimately, this explains the importance of utilizing culinary arts in your journey through grief. Cooking-for-one is a difficult step to take, but one that brings us closer to the continuous bond between ourselves and those we have lost. All of us want to feel closer to our loved ones, honor them, and remember them proudly. With culinary grief therapy, we accomplish just that.

CHAPTER 7

Guided Recipe Memoir Writing

As already discussed, journaling is a very healthy coping strategy in grief and loss. However, it may be difficult at times to just write. Therefore, it is helpful to have a prompt or tool to work from.

A powerful tool in grief work is guided memoir writing using recipes as your guide. The goal here is to integrate the loss by telling a memorable story without having it feel like a writing assignment. When you process your experience this way, the story itself takes your writing to places you never thought it would go and reminds you of special memories tucked safely away.

To reach this state of writing, we can use recipes as memoirs. With every recipe, there is always a story. For example, as think you of a familiar recipe, consider the following:

- Where did you have the meal?
- Who was with you?
- What was the season?
- What was the conversation?
- What was the occasion?
- What were the feelings?
- What was the weather like?
- What did the food smell and taste like?

Use recipes to help you journal and reflect on special memories to heal you on your journey. In thinking of recipes, be sure not to think too literally. Let the recipes and stories come naturally. You do not have to use complete, elaborate recipes. In fact, the simple ones sometimes mean more. For example, when you think of your loved one's favorite summer recipe, it can be as simple as the following:

- Burger [cooked medium]
  Think of how your loved one preferred his or her meat cooked. Use specific details.
- Bun [sesame seed always]
  Think if your loved one was particular with a type of burger bun or brand.
- Cheese [cheddar cheese always]

> Do not leave out any details. Reflect on all the specifics as if he or she was ordering or cooking right in front of you. Capture a memory.

Once you have the details, write the story. Let the cooking, smell, and meal guide you in your writing so that you can share those memories you hold so dearly. The more you think of the meals and focus on the smell of the cooking, the more stories and memories will begin to appear. Write down all the thoughts that come to mind. Do not worry about putting sentences in chronological order—just write. Afterward you can go back and rephrase or realign. Just get it all out while you are taken back in time.

Guided Memoir-Writing Exercise

What was your loved one's favorite ______________________________ recipe?

Where did you have the meal?

Who was with you?

When was the meal?

Why was the meal prepared? What was the occasion?

How was the conversation? What was discussed?

What did the food smell and taste like?

What was the weather like on that day?

What feelings were experienced on that day?

Why did your loved one say this was his or her favorite recipe?

What do you remember most about your loved one with this recipe?

How does this recipe make you feel?

Share a favorite memory of your loved one in relation to the recipe chosen.

Personal-Reflection Exercise

How do I feel when I think of cooking-for-one?

How do I react when I walk into the kitchen?

How do I react when I walk into the grocery store?

What mealtime is the most difficult for me? Why?

What task, activity, or program can I participate in during mealtimes?

What recipe would I like to try in the future? (If nothing comes to mind, take a few minutes to explore recipes in books, on the Internet, or at home.)

What strengths have I discovered that I never knew I had?

What do I fear the most about cooking-for-one?

What do I feel hopeful or joyous about in trying to cook-for-one?

What is my meaning for cooking today? What do I want to accomplish with my cooking today?

If I were to prepare a simple meal for my loved one today, what would I prepare?
Active coping technique: prepare the meal, and then journal the experience.

How do I feel today?

How can I reward myself for going to the grocery store or cooking a meal-for-one? Identify multiple ways.

What do I want to tell myself on this journey?

Trigger-Identification Exercise

A grief trigger is any stimulus that brings up memories related to a loss. Triggers may be obvious and easy to anticipate, but many are spontaneous and come without warning. You can think of grief triggers as mines in a minefield. Each day you try to make your way carefully through a maze you have no map for, knowing a mine can go off at any time.

An important part of the journey of grief work is identifying previously experienced triggers and practicing healthy coping strategies for the unidentified ones. Use the exercise below to help you with trigger identification.

What are some of your identified grief triggers? Write down those previously experienced.

What are some unidentified triggers you have experienced? Write down those that were spontaneous.

How do you take care of yourself after a trigger (or how would you like to)?

Do you prefer to talk to someone after a trigger or rather participate in a task or project?

Create a list of things that produce a strong wave of grief for you. This could include a car, a store, a restaurant, a song, a scent, a doctor, or a room, to name a few. Think of situations that have occurred in which you experienced strong waves of grief. Also think of situations that might produce a strong wave in the future. Take a couple of moments to visually walk through a few days in your head, and notice any heightened reactions.

Reflect upon your relationship to the grief trigger. Then write a letter or note to your loved one and discuss the trigger in order to process the experience for healing.
What do you want to say in this present moment regarding the grief trigger you experienced?

CHAPTER 8

Recipes for My Journey

Consider using your own recipes for the different themes and seasons previously discussed to reflect upon your personal journey.

Recipe for the Days You Cannot Get Out of Bed or Stop the Tears

Recipe for Eating Outdoors to Catch Some Fresh Air

Recipe for Lifting Your Spirits

Recipe for the Good Days

Recipe for the Bad Days

Recipe for Grieving during the Holidays

Recipe for the Fall

Recipe for the Winter

Recipe for the Spring

Recipe for the Summer

Recipe for Birthdays

Recipe to Reward Yourself and Recognize Your Strengths

Recipe that Inspired You from a Cooking-for-One Workshop or Life Experience

Recipe that You Loved Cooking for Your Loved One or Your Loved One Loved Cooking for You

Recipes for My Journey

Recipes for My Journey

Recipes for My Journey

Recipes for My Journey

Recipes for My Journey

Recipes for My Journey

Recipes for My Journey

Afterword

For more information on *Culinary Grief Therapy: Cooking-for-One* workshops or to register for a series contact Heather Lynn Nickrand, MA, LPC, NCC, Bereavement Coordinator of AMITA Health Alexian Brothers Hospice.

Heather L. Nickrand, MA, LPC, NCC
Hospice Bereavement Coordinator
Hospice Volunteer Supervisor

AMITA HEALTH

Alexian Brothers Hospice
1515 E. Lake Street, Suite 206
Hanover Park, IL 60133
630.233.5100 o
630.233.5118 d
630.233.5101 f
heather.nickrand@AMITAhealth.org

AMITAhealth.org

Made in the USA
Monee, IL
01 December 2021

83521299R10048